PATHWAYS:

Discovering the Power Within

A TESTIMONY OF GOD BREAKING FOOD ADDICTIONS

BY: YOLANDA FLEMING-WILLIAMS

Copyright © 2020 Yolanda Fleming-Williams

All rights reserved, including the right to reproduce this book or portions thereof in any form whatsoever by author. No part of this book may be reproduced, scanned or distributed in any print or electric form without author's prior express written consent. Please do not participate or encourage piracy of copyrighted materials in violation of author's rights.

This is a work of fiction. Names, characters, businesses, places, events, locales, and incidents are either the products of the author's imagination or used in a fictitious manner. Any resemblance to actual persons, living or dead, or actual events is purely coincidental.

Scripture quotations are taken from the Holy Bible. King James Version

ISBN: 978-1-7353541-2-5

Published by: Writing in Faith

Baton Rouge, La.

IAMWRITINGINFAITH.COM

Cover design by Aaron Mcbride/ radiancegraphics@gmail.com

Editing by Alecia Rhoe/ rhoe9891@gmail.com

Photography by Peter G. Forest/ www.forestphotollc.com

For more information address:

Attention Yolanda Fleming-Williams at Yolawilliams40@gmail.com

Yolanda Fleming-Williams (text)

PATHWAYS-Discovering The Power Within

TABLE OF CONTENTS

Dedication ....

Introduction: Allowing Full Access ....

Acknowledgements ....

Chapter 1: When We First Met 1

Chapter 2: To Obey or Not to Obey..5

Chapter 3: Special Delivery..9

Chapter 4: Unwanted Interruption..13

Chapter 5: Inspire One..19

Chapter 6: Let's Get There! I Encourage You.....................................25

Intercessory Prayer of New Life...29

Author Contact Page...

DEDICATION

This book is dedicated to my beloved big brother, Antonio Fleming, also known as,

"Cool Tony, Winner of War."

Rest in peace, my sweet brother.

INTRODUCTION: ALLOWING FULL ACCESS

The Holy Spirit is always there, willing and ready to change us; however, we must surrender all unto Him by allowing Him access to every door of our lives. Once this takes place, He can begin to reveal the changes that must be made. He can clean areas in our lives that are just, plain dirty, and touch areas that may need healing. We must realize it is a process and nothing will happen overnight, over a week, or even a month's time. We must allow Him full access to the cabinets of our hearts, mind, and soul.

Let's start with how thoughts enter our minds. Our ears are open to polluted conversations. Therefore, we must be mindful of what we listen to outside of the Word of God. Faith comes by hearing, and hearing God's Word. In order to keep our minds free and unpolluted, we must stay away from any form of ungodly communication.

Whether it is close friends or even family, set a standard for yourself and for them. Be bold in saying that you no longer want to hear gossip or the latest hearsay, which may result in your separation from certain activities or events. This must be done in an effort to keep your mind free and clear of any disturbances. Peace of mind is your target. Your soul is the innermost place where everything dwells. It is where everything is stored: happiness, hurts, confusion, disappointments, rejections, bruises, and thorns-the good and bad. Within our soul lies our beliefs, unbelief, treasures, forgiveness, and unforgiveness. We must allow the Holy Spirit to console and mend our soul, to cover and heal all the bruises and every bad thing that has ever happened in our lives, including the pains from childhood memories.

Maybe you saw fights between your parents and those memories still taunt you, causing you to have a bad outlook or approach concerning dating and marriage. Maybe you were teased as a child in school, and it has affected your social skills as an adult. You may find it hard to trust people and build meaningful relationships. We must remember that the Holy Spirit was given to us as a gift, not to be put on a shelf. The Holy Spirit is a gift, that when given total access, brings forth change in our lives. We must allow Him in, so He can access all these negative accounts in our lives and begin to build positive ones. After allowing the Holy Spirit all access and totally surrendering our lives letting Him heal our souls, and all the bruises from the past, then we can concentrate and move on to the heart.

With the heart, man believes unto righteousness. You see, it is our hearts that must be healthy, but we cannot have a healthy heart if our soul is still carrying bruises and hurts from our past. Once our souls are healed totally by the Holy Spirit of God, we must believe again, and I mean *truly believe*. We must believe we can trust again, believe we can love again, and believe we can totally forgive every negative action and person of our past. Then the heart is ready to be open once more: open to love, trust, and forgive. Afterwards, because the soul is healed, there is peace again, which is the peace of God that surpasses all understanding, which now enables you to live a righteous, holy, and healthy life.

You can live a life that is totally dependent on God, and you can begin to master the Fruit of the Spirit and live freely with true godliness. We know that the Fruit of the Spirit is love, joy, peace, longsuffering, gentleness, goodness, faith, meekness, and temperance. Against these, there is nothing. So, allow the Spirit to give you back your passion for life, and begin to say "yes" to life, love, and relationships. Peace and the full, goodness of life are your targets and the Holy Spirit can get you there. There is no limit to what God can do for you!

ACKNOWLEDGEMENTS

I would like to thank God for all of His wonderful blessings: my husband Ray, my children, and my entire family. I'm forever grateful for Your love and patience.

~ Chapter 1 ~

When We First Met

When I think back to my childhood days, I have always had an issue with one of the biggest things we need in life to survive and that is food! It's not that I had a bad childhood and would look to food for comfort. In fact, I have fond memories of my early days as a child. Mom always made sure we had a cooked breakfast—cereal occasionally. And Dad? Well, before I entered school, he worked nights, so I hung out with him most of the day. We would ride to my grandmother's house every morning, and on the way to her house was this little, silver building that sold the best donuts in the world.

As a little four-year-old girl, every morning, I would tell Dad to *please* get me one glazed and one chocolate donut, and a chocolate milk. Did I say every morning? Yes, I did! I had to have both donuts, simply because I needed to know which one was better. Although I knew that both would be delicious, I just had to have them both. After getting my favorite donuts, we would head to my grandmother's house and you know the first thing she would ask me was, "Are you hungry? Did you have something to eat, yet?" And before I could answer, she had already began preparing my plate. There was no way I could turn her food down and possibly hurt her feelings, could I? So, I accepted my food and carried on.

Little did I know, this food habit would haunt me for the next 40 years. Now as an adult, I can see that same pattern with food. When it is time to choose between two different kinds of meat or bread, I still want them both just to compare which one tastes better. I would ask myself, why couldn't I have just enough discipline to choose one over the other, and be satisfied? In this book you will discover ways to discipline yourself when making food choices, how to gain self-control over bad eating habits, and how to love yourself during the entire process.

I can remember Friday nights, especially. I was about nine or ten years old. We would have fried chicken, and it was my Mama's fried chicken, if you know what I mean. *Down south folk know exactly what I mean!* Anyway, we had that fried chicken, red beans, biscuits, and shrimp fried rice. Dad would bring home that delicious, lemon meringue pie from McKenzie. Man, oh man! I couldn't wait for Friday nights! I wanted the biggest piece of that chicken, which was the breast of course, and it would be mine, skin and all, along with all the fixings—which I enjoyed. Little did I know, those same exact foods would be my worst enemy, today.

I think back to how my gluttonous habits began. Instead of one sandwich, I would have two. I would sneak pies to my room. My mom would see me with one, but I would secretly have another tucked away in my shirt. Does that sound funny or familiar? This was the beginning of a horrible trap; at least for me, it was. I was always on a journey with food, which resembled an up and down roller coaster ride. The spirit of gluttony played a major role in my life because I wanted two or more of everything. *Wow!*

Later, as I entered high school, I developed a habit of not eating breakfast or lunch. I would eat when I got home, but I overindulged when eating. For instance, I would get a sandwich, a snack, and then eat whatever meal my mom prepared. And, yes, even after this I would eat, again. I was young at the time, so being that my metabolism was still working properly, my weight or sickness really was not the problem, so in my mind I was fine. I didn't realize that I was headed down a very unhealthy path by continuing in such an undisciplined lifestyle with food.

After high school, I gave birth to my first son. After having him, I decided to join the Navy. In joining the Navy, I knew I needed to diet and exercise. My mind was set to succeed in this lifechanging goal, so I chose to try a new diet. I took a load of pills that were designed to quickly shape up my body and get me ready to move. The next three months it was me, exercise, and this diet program. This diet program worked during the time of my life in the military. My eating habits weren't too bad because I was always busy working or hanging out with my friends, although I'd simultaneously entered an unhealthy relationship.

After entering this relationship, my eating habits began to become unhealthy once more. I can remember during this time in my life when my harmful eating habits would return and stick around for a while, causing high blood pressure, diabetes, sleep apnea, and cardiomegaly. To be brutally honest, even though I had received these diagnoses from the doctors, I still ate what I wanted when I wanted. My doctors would tell me, "Miss Williams, we believe you suffer from binge eating," and I was like "What?!"

At times I would crave sweets, like candy, cake, and ice cream. Yeah, I'm calling all my enemies out! I would lose weight, eating right and exercising, then something would cause me to lose focus and I would get into this uncontrollable fight with food. It was crazy. For about three months straight, I would eat my favorite candies, pizza, burgers, chips, and fries. You name it, I ate it. I would be in this horrible place, then the cravings would eventually slow down, and I would start back to some type of health diet.

I have done almost every diet pill out there, so I know the daily struggle of wanting to do better with your health and eating properly, while saying to yourself, "Today is the day!" You do good the first couple of days, and boom, it's 'so and so's' birthday, and the cycle starts all over again.

After some time passed during these cycles, I had gotten married and had two more sons. I can remember a time when my sons were younger, and I would go grocery shopping and buy these cookies out of the store. I would buy two packs: one entire pack for myself to eat and the replacement pack. *Come on. Don't laugh.* Somebody out there can relate. What? Did I not think the weight was going to show on me? Do you see how blinded I was by the spirit of gluttony? These are the types of things that continued until I was diagnosed with diabetes from eating too much sugar, making me feel horrible and causing my body to act strangely.

In 2016, some friends shared with me about a high protein diet that would change my life, so I decided to try it, and yes, it changed my life. I lost so many inches and pounds, and I was very, proud of myself. I felt this was the one miracle diet I had been waiting for, although it was just a year after that I had gained almost all the weight back. Because of the weight gain, I had to get back on the medications, which I said I would never return to.

∼ Chapter 2 ∼

To Obey or Not to Obey

Now, the true journey begins with just me here in a decision-making place. The question is, do I want to live my life being controlled by bad food cravings and gluttony, or do I want to utilize the God-given gift of the Holy Spirit to rescue me? In utilizing this power, I will receive guidance on how to gain the discipline and authority I need to conquer and win this battle against bad food cravings. The Bible says that Jesus left us the Holy Spirit as a Comforter, a Teacher, and a Guide. We must begin to use the gift of the Holy Spirit, by allowing Him to guide, lead, and help us make the right decisions, even concerning food. We cannot allow food to dominate us. When we do not utilize the Holy Spirit, I believe we grieve Him. He is waiting for us to grab hold, so that He can propel us into our next level.

So, my question to those of you reading this book is this: Are you ready just say; *"I USED TO BE?"*

We will begin with love. Loving God says, *I love God and He loves me.* Yes, God loves us all. John 3:16 says, "For God so loved the world, that He gave His only begotten Son…"—His only unique Son—that if we believe and trust in Him, we're going to have eternal, everlasting life. We often see this scripture being used along with the teachings for salvation and having new life in Christ. True, it goes well with that scripture, but if we read it again, it can also be used in other aspects of our Christian life. God loves us so much that He gave something He loved dearly. He sacrificed His only Son, His only unique Son, so that we would not perish, but would have eternal and everlasting life.

When I think about the word perish, I think of suffering, whether suffering death suddenly or in an untimely way. All I could think about was the fact that, in a moment I could suddenly die in an untimely way. If I say I'm a believer and believe He [God] left me a comforter and teacher to help me, but I don't utilize the gift of the Holy Spirit, then all He has done would be in vain. As stated before, this grieves Him, and I thought to myself, I don't want to grieve the Holy Spirit or disappoint God. With this in mind, I am striving to please God with my eating habits because I want Him to be proud of me. I want Him to be pleased with who He created me to be.

I have been speaking to myself for several months on how I was going to get my breakthrough. Keep in mind, I was still struggling with the bad food habits, but I kept at it almost every day. If I didn't say it aloud, I thought it and remembered the Bible saying in Proverbs 18:21, "Death and life are in the power of the tongue." It is very, important that, even if we have not reached our goal, we continue to listen and confess it.

I can remember being at my mom's house, and we were all talking and laughing. Amidst this, a fast food commercial played, advertising a double cheeseburger and tots for about $2.00. I think my eyes immediately set gaze on it, until I could literally taste it. I can also remember wanting a chocolate shake to go along with it. On my way to get my son from work that day, I stopped at that fast food restaurant, and ordered exactly what I saw and desired. As I sat there, immediately my Helper, the Holy Spirit said, "You don't need that; you know what it's going to do to you. Think about it. Think about the consequences and the effects this will have on you."

I fought with the temptation for about a good five minutes and it was hard, but I said, "No." I backed out of that fast food restaurant parking lot and did not look back. I wanted what I wanted but realized that what was bad or evil for me was not going to add any goodness to my life or my body. In Matthew chapter 6, verses 22 to 23 it says, *"The light of the body is the eye: if therefore thine eye be single, thy whole body shall be full of light. But if thine eye be evil, thy whole body shall be full of darkness. If therefore the light that is in thee be darkness, how great is that darkness?"*

It is so important that we guard ourselves from what we see or how we see things. Therefore, I am now careful regarding these things. I pray and ask the Holy Spirit to help me in these areas. Another person may see the same commercial, and just see a fast food advertisement, without it becoming a temptation for them. For someone like me, on the other hand, who deals with issues and temptations such as the spirit of gluttony, it is a very, different situation. If I'm not prayed up, I see opportunity to give into temptation and fall back into my old habits of eating.

We must keep God ever before us, always meditating on His word. One powerful scripture to meditate on is Philippians 3:19 (NIV). It says, "Their destiny is destruction, their god is their stomach, and their glory is in their shame. Their mind is on earthly things." We don't want to shame God, when we know He has given us the gift of the Holy Spirit to help us in every area possible.

I believe what we all can learn through this entire process is the ability to fall in love with God and love ourselves where we are currently. If you can get through an hour without overeating, overindulging, or choosing something unhealthy, you should reward yourself by saying something great and positive about yourself. If that hour alone is a great success, that one hour of success has the capability to give you the power to conquer the entire day. You can go back and reflect and say, *If I can get through one hour, I'm going to get through the next hour*, and now your strength begins to develop, and it makes you stronger every day. You can begin to look forward to a brighter tomorrow.

During this process, I had to reunite with the truth, which was, God loves me so much that I can overcome anything trying to attack and destroy me, by the power of God, through my faith in Him. I now realize why Jesus came to set us free from any demonic force that would try to destroy His purpose and plan for our lives. Jesus' coming means *nothing* and *no one* can conquer or destroy us because of God's word. We are more than conquerors through Christ Jesus, our Lord!

Chapter 3

Special Delivery

Now at this point, it is time to get focused and disciplined. It is time to gain back control over our bad food habits and over gluttony. I know you are asking, *'How do I accomplish this?'* You are probably saying, *'I've tried every method known to man'*, as we all may say at one point in our lives. Now is the time to totally depend on God for the strength and support you will need. This is the difference, this time around. It will be total dependence on God, not trying to do it with your own strength, like all the other times before.

Yes, I'm guilty of trying everything else at one point in my life. I thought it was up to others to help encourage me, to stop me from choosing the wrong foods to eat or even giving me the right portions. I was counting on my family to help me, but that was not always the case. They are all healthy and they eat how they want, and when they want. So, most of time I found I was in this battle alone physically, although spiritually, I found what and who I really needed. I needed discipline. I needed the power of the Holy Spirit to teach me how to choose the right foods and lead me in how to use portion control. I believe we all need to gain this type of discipline, not only with food, but with anything we are battling in our lives or that is hindering us from having success in our lives.

I can recall being in the supermarket one day and seeing an older lady I knew. She shared with me how she was a compulsive buyer, and how she would want things out of the store that she really didn't need. She shared how it used to be a big problem for her. She then expressed how, when shopping in the store, she now goes down the aisles, asking the Holy Spirit to guide her and to keep her from overspending on things she really doesn't need. I remembered all the things that she told me and later decided to try this approach with the way I was abusing food. Sure, I know I need food for energy and nutrition, but it's up to me to choose the right types of food and the correct portions, right?

We must encourage ourselves. God has already given us the authority over everything, so we don't have any excuses not to succeed in this life. God has given us everything pertaining to life and godliness, and He does not want us hurting ourselves with anything, certainly not food. Many of the foods today are very unhealthy for us, especially those loaded with sugar and salt. We must find ways to conquer these cravings for these foods. I have learned to stop looking to just eat for the taste or flavor, and I try to enjoy the goodness of food for the nutrition and energy. Even though I was still choosing and eating poorly, I would say to myself out loud, today is my day to get my eating habits right with God. I had to speak what I wanted to see every day. Am I done? Absolutely not! It's a daily choice between what's available now and what I can discipline myself to wait on that will benefit me, and please God at the same time.

First Corinthians chapter 9 and verse 27 (ESV) says, "But I discipline my body and bring it into subjection, lest after preaching to others, I myself should be disqualified." I want to do what I do for myself, to become better so that I might work for God in His kingdom. However, if I don't practice what I'm delivering to others, how can I be a benefit to God's kingdom or His people? This simply means, I must communicate daily with God by submitting myself totally to Him and allowing His power to overtake me when temptation comes.

James chapter 4 and verse 7 (NIV) says, "Submit yourselves, then, to God. Resist the devil and he will flee from you." Once we submit to God, the Holy Spirit will come and remind us of our confessions concerning our lives and eating habits, then strength will come, and we will conquer in that hour and hours to come. Romans chapter 8 and verse 37 (NIV) says, "No, in all these things we are more than conquerors through him that loved us." All of this brings me here: the state where I am today. I am more conscious of what I ingest because now I ask myself, am I pleasing God? One of my greatest temptations is the desire for the taste of what is forbidden—the strength of not reacting to impulse. I am still in the process of disciplining myself, as stated before; it is a daily walk. My goal is to desire and crave God like I used to desire and crave those foods, to use that same energy I used for food, and put it into my love and my desire for God. This story will never end. It will only get better as I continue to obey God's voice and live out my purpose and my destiny.

Yolanda Fleming-Williams

Chapter 4

Unwanted Interruption

Just when I thought I was good and had it "down packed" as they say, the dreadful day came right in the middle of writing this book. I fell off *the truck, the ladder*, and *anything else* you can fall off. I can't tell you how or exactly when, but the wellness coach fell back into her old eating habits. I got stressed about life and one day temptation came, and I allowed this flesh to temporarily win. The bad cravings came back to haunt me. I asked myself, *Why?* And why in the middle of my book? I thought, *oh my God! I'm supposed to be a leader, an example.* I feared not being able to get back on track. I thought to myself, how could I now make videos concerning this? Then I heard, *love yourself where you are and begin again. It's okay.* I thought to myself, *Yes, I'm still a leader, and yes Lord, I can still be Your example.*

You know love is such a powerful word. Love mends together everything that is broken. Love creates not just children, but it creates beautiful art, lovely songs, and long-lasting relationships. We smile out of love. We are patient because of love. Love makes us grow. Love makes us communicate. Love makes us forgive. Because of love, we hope and dream. Love makes us successful. Because of love, we received a gift, and not just any gift. Love gave us new life. By all means, don't take this as just a cliché, but love really is the key, and Jesus is love.

So, you ask what did I do? Simple: whenever it came up on me, I began to tell myself, *I love you Yolanda. You're special to me, and no, this journey is not easy, but it's your journey. I am designed especially for it. I will overcome my temptations day by day, sometimes minute by minute.* I have realized that I am in charge and with the Holy Spirit, I can and do all things through Christ who strengthens me.

Every day I thank God through praise and worship. I thank Him for His anointing, for His grace is sufficient and His mercy is brand new every day. I give Him honor and glory because it all belongs to Him. I found that on this journey of mine, I still had hidden issues from the past, buried deep in my soul. Twenty years of marriage to my wonderful husband, no infidelity to acknowledge, and I still had trust issues. He and I both thought that maybe the key for me was being set free, dealing with why I had trust issues even with him and he did nothing wrong.

Neither of us are perfect. We have heated fellowship like everyone else, but for the most part we grow and get over it. Through talking one day, he opened up and shared with me a concern of his. He said to me, throughout all the years we have been together, he felt I never trusted him totally with my heart, and that I may not admit it. He knew that I didn't because of walls that I have built inside. He talked for about 15 minutes. I was very, very still and quiet. In fact, I was speechless. I could not say a word because he had hit it on the nose, or as we say *bullseye*. I thought to myself, *this man of mine*. It was evening time, and he was leaving for work. I had no plans, but I knew I needed to write.

Did I feel like writing? No. So, I took a nap that evening and there it was again: *write*! Write! So, I began to drill myself. *Why do I have trust issues with a man who loves me unconditionally, by God's grace? What am I afraid of? What do I not want to face?* Those were my questions to myself. That night was a true turning point in my life and my marriage. I didn't run from his concerns; I was open, honest, and vulnerable.

When we met over 20 years ago, I had already had a child—that's pretty much all he knew. I didn't discuss my past much. At 17, I became pregnant. When I graduated high school, I was already 4 and ½ to 5 months pregnant, and still in denial. I was terrified to tell my parents, especially my dad, knowing the disappointment I would have to face. I knew I couldn't keep it a secret much longer. Finally, after graduation, the truth came out, but God was in the midst. I remember Him sending a very, nice librarian to my life who helped me get to the point where I could tell my parents; she was there with me every step of the way. *Thanks Miss Hall*.

The situation was not easy after telling my parents. Of course they wanted to see what the other side had to say. Let's just say for book purposes, I'll stay nice and simple. Not that my parents were trying to marry me off, they just wanted to know the intentions of taking care of responsibilities, but at that time, it wasn't very pleasant. What's a 17 years old girl to do? *Move on!* And that's what I did, concentrating on me and my baby I would be having. For the next six months, I got to know how loving and forgiving my parents were. They became my rock through it all, especially my mother. I didn't worry about what so-called friends were saying. I was just enjoying what my parents were doing for me, as we prepared for this new life that was coming very quickly.

I believe I truly needed all that love and support to carry me through—love from Mom and Dad, and the rest of my family and friends. You see, I had buried my true feelings about how I felt about the rejection and betrayal I felt from the other side. By saying I moved on, I did just that; I moved on. I didn't pack up and leave it. I hide it deep inside, hoping it would never return, meaning my feelings of betrayal, hurt, rejection, and disappointment really didn't get acknowledged. Trust was broken, and I didn't deal with it.

I was 17. Who knows how to deal with anything at 17? All those feelings were just left somewhere, not acknowledged—somewhere in the chamber of my soul. Now, over 20 years, three more kids, and a dog later, I must deal with this magnitude of a situation. In those days, it was quite devastating to me, but with God, I made it through a tough time. Outwardly, I managed to get through with a smile. My mom and dad worked every day, so of course I was home alone with the dog and a TV I didn't watch much. Most of the time I was alone during the day, and most days I found myself calling the young man asking him why is he lying and slandering my name, when he knew it was only me and him, but at 17 who wants the responsibility of being a parent? However, to have my name slandered, and to be lied about bothered me a lot, but what could I do?

I eventually left the situation alone with the young man. I started concentrating on me and my most precious gift: my son. Now I'm here, 27 years later realizing what I hadn't dealt with at 17. At 17, my mind was not able to deal with something as major as this kind of hurt, rejection, and broken trust. Now, here I am at 45, married for over 20 years, with four children. It is not that I have hate or dislike in my heart; truly I don't. No, I didn't like the way things were handled and I can't base that one incident on how others will treat me. I must learn, and have learned, to give everyone the benefit of the doubt. Now, what's next after 27 years after finding out I must go back and deal with some feelings from my past that I didn't know how to deal with at that time. I have done the first thing, which is I realized it. I faced it!

I worked my way through it and benefited from it. This life is truly a work-in-progress. Who knew something I experienced over 27 years ago had affected me, my relationships, and my thought process when it came to allowing myself to be free enough to love freely? I thank God that I'm taking control today, finding the peace I need in order to truly move on from past hurts. Now I can live the life God truly intended for me to live in my marriage and as a mother, because the worst thing we can do is pass these things onto our children.

Learning to trust again brought on a new meaning of love, and this process doesn't happen overnight. It takes time to allow old wounds to heal. We can't rush it and we also can't allow it to dictate our future. We must allow God to give us what we need so that we can conqueror fears, hurts, disappointments, and rejection. Little did I know, those hidden feelings were controlling me even as far as my eating habits. I wasn't designed to be an overeater, but if we don't search ourselves daily, we will end up being something that God did not ordain us to be. Don't be afraid to go back and search within yourself and find the hidden hurts, rejections, and sadness. Begin to work on them so that you can live and be free, living the life that God intended for you to live.

God bless and remember *love yourself where you are.*

⁴*Love is patient, love is kind. It does not envy, it does not boast, it is not proud.*

⁵ *It does not dishonor others, it is not self-seeking, it is not easily angered, it keeps no record of wrongs.*

⁶ *Love does not delight in evil but rejoices with the truth.*

⁷ *It always protects, always trusts, always hopes, always perseveres.*

⁸ *Love never fails...*

꙳1 Corinthians 13: 4-8 (NIV)꙳

ALL THINGS ARE POSSIBLE WITH GOD!!

∼ Chapter 5 ∼

Inspire One

Inspirational Quotes

The words we speak have power. We can speak life or death to a person or a situation. Watch the words that come out of your mouth, because you never know what is on a person's mind or what they are facing. Someone may be on the edge of giving up and your one word, phrase, or even your attitude could change their life and change their future.

Being mindful of the words that we use is one of the purposes of my ministry, Christ Producing Restoration Ministries, which social media page can be found on Facebook. As you take this journey and become more aware of how you speak about yourself and others, I encourage you to use the hashtag *#CPR,* for *Christ Producing Restoration,* as a reminder that it is because of Him that you are able to see change. Use the preceding hashtag on your social media sites when speaking about your life's journey toward health and wellness.

Below are inspirational quotes inspired by the Holy Spirit through scriptural referencing, as well as through general revelation of this journey.

Watch your mouth.

Proverbs 18:21 (KJV): "Death and life are in the power of the tongue…"

Be beneficial, not a beneficiary; you might not want what you inherit.

Comfort one another.

1 Thessalonians 5:11 (KJV): "Wherefore comfort yourselves together, and edify one another, even as also ye do."

Don't just seek a gift, be a gift.

Wrap yourself in Him.

Romans 12:1 (NIV): "Therefore, I urge you, brothers and sisters, in view of God's mercy, to offer your bodies a living sacrifice, holy and pleasing to God—this is your true and proper worship."

We all would be smart if only we had understanding.

#keepPEACEalive

Proverbs 4:7 (KJV): "Wisdom is the principal thing; therefore get wisdom: and with all thy getting get understanding."

When you find out God loves you, no more sad days.

Jeremiah 29:11 (AMP): "For I know the plans and thoughts that I have for you, says the Lord, plans for peace and well-being and not for disaster, to give you a future and a hope."

Birds sing. Flowers bloom. Trees shed. What are you doing?

#movesomething

James 2:20 (KJV): "But wilt thou know, O vain man, that faith without works is dead?"

Sometimes, you must slow down, and reflect on that day when you first met Jesus.

Oh, what a time!

Matthew 18:11 (KJV): "For the Son of man is come to save that which was lost."

Don't ignore the call with foolish living.

Imitate God.

John 4:28-29 (KJV): "The woman that left her waterpot, and went her way into the city, and saith to the men, 'Come, see a man, which told me all things that I ever did: is not this the Christ?"

Don't just have power, give power. Be a witness; testify the goodness.

1 Timothy 4:14 (KJV): "Neglect not the gift that is in thee, which was given thee by prophecy, with the laying on of the hands of the presbytery."

Luke 14:23 (KJV): "And the lord said unto the servant, Go out into the highways and hedges, and compel them to come in, that my house may be filled."

To be a good writer, you must be a good listener. To be a good listener, you must be a good teacher. To be a good teacher, you must be a good illustrator. To be a good illustrator, you must be a good student.

Regenerate yourself; be used by Him.

2nd Timothy 2:15 (KJV): "Study to shew thyself approved unto God, a workman that needeth not to be ashamed, rightly dividing the word of truth."

Be excited for what God is sending your way.

#expectation

Philippians 4:6 (NIV): "Do not be anxious about anything, but in every situation, by prayer and petition, with thanksgiving, present your requests to God."

You can't control what a person says or think about you.

Live life pleasing God.

Philippians 4:7 (KJV): "And the peace of God, which passeth all understanding, shall keep your hearts and minds through Christ Jesus."

So what, we don't sometimes understand why certain things happen in our lives? Why things don't go as planned? It may be a good thing, but God knows what is best. He knows what's ahead. He keeps us from harm and danger.

Protector. Deliverer. Always on time.

Genesis 22:14 (KJV): "And Abraham called the name of that place Jehovah-jireh: as it is said to this day, in the mount of the Lord it shall be seen."

Don't mumble and complain; be grateful. It could be worse.

#BeContent #BeJoyful

Philippians 2:14 (KJV): "Do all things without murmurings and disputings:"

With my whole heart I believe whatever I ask according to the will of God I shall have.

#repeat #receive

John 14:13-14 (NIV): "And I will do whatever you ask in my name, so that the Father may be glorified in the Son. You may ask me for anything in my name, and I will do it."

God is good in all seasons.

#testify #heNEVERchanges

Hebrews 13:8 (NIV): "Jesus Christ is the same yesterday and today and forever."

Sometimes you just have to smile in the depths of trouble, no matter what.

James 1:2-4 (KJV): "My brethren, count it all joy when ye fall into divers temptations; knowing this, that the trying of your faith worketh patience. But let patience have her perfect work, that ye may be perfect and entire, wanting nothing."

Chapter 6

Let's Get There! I Encourage You!

It's time now to fall in love with God, love yourself where you are, be obedient to the Holy Spirit, and study the Word. Do everything in moderation. Allow the Word of God to restore you. Choose to be disciplined by the Word of God, daily. We are in this together. I am believing that God will enlighten you on what He wants you to do regarding developing healthy eating habits. Just sit still and listen to Him; He will teach you how to make the right choices in every area of life. Again, begin with an open heart, and a renewed mind. Do this by inviting God into your heart. My hope is that you will find the treasure you have hidden inside of yourself. It's not hard when you have God involved. Having God makes it easy. God says in His word that we should take on His yoke and learn of Him, because His yoke is easy, and His burden is light. Be blessed and enjoy your journey.

LET'S GET STARTED

Journal Daily

Describe any issues you may have had— past or present—that may contribute to negative food habits and choices. _____

_____

_____
_____
_____
_____

List any hurts you need to release.

_____
_____
_____
_____
_____
_____

If you have anyone you need to forgive, ask God to show you how and what to exercise daily:

- Meditate

- If you don't have one, get a hobby

- Do something new everyday

- List your daily successes

- List any challenges of the day or week

Here are six, healthy tips inspired by the Holy Spirit, that will help you on your journey towards health and wellness.

1. **Eat to satisfy**.

    You will know when you are full. Listen to your body and begin to accept what your body is saying. It's all in your mind. So, enjoy your food, but think about what you're eating. Ask yourself, *will this meal produce good results— not only on the outside, but on the inside, as well?* Be conscious and thoughtful when preparing your meals.

2. **Chewing is very, important**.

    Take your time and again enjoy your food: the smell and the taste. Think about being full and satisfied. Build a healthy relationship with your food. Remember that you're the only person that knows the needs of your body, especially when it comes to your health and wellness.

3. **Water, water, and yes, more water.**

    Water is the key. The more you drink, the more hydrated your body becomes. Water aides in our digestion of food and it helps in our feelings of being full and satisfied. Try drinking a glass before and after each meal.

4. **Try to eat small meals during the day.**

    Choose foods that will nourish your mind, body, and soul, like fruits or your favorite vegetables. When on the go, first think about what you're going to eat. Plan your meals and snacks ahead of time.

5. **Again, choose foods that will promote healing within your body.**

    Remember, your body is the temple of the Holy Spirit, so be mindful of what you feed your spirit.

6. **Last, but not least, turn off all distractions.**

    That includes T.V., radio, and the cell phone. Repeat after me: "No social media while eating." Give your meals your undivided attention. Enjoy the aroma and savor the taste, and I promise you will be full and satisfied.

～ Intercessory Prayer for New Life ～

The enemy is trying to attack God's children with many sicknesses and diseases, but I am calling every prayer warrior — every intercessor — to pray this prayer.

To those who are suffering with unknown causes of pain and all forms of cancers, blood clots, cataracts, brain disorders, HIV/ AIDS, Alzheimer's, ADHD, arthritis, any kind of autoimmune diseases, CROHN'S disease, GRAVES disease, glaucoma, diabetes and everything associated with it, depression and everything associated with it, fibromyalgia, GERD, GOUT, hepatitis, high blood pressure, headaches, insomnia, kidney disease, mental illness, MS, heart attacks, hip and knee replacements, PTSD, seizures, sickle cell, sleep apnea, stress, strokes, tumors and any kind of ungodly, unhealthy addictions: BE HEALED IN THE NAME OF JESUS!

No more premature deaths. Move by Your Spirit, Lord!

In Jesus' name, Amen.

We need each other. Therefore, let us agree in prayer every day, but on today, let us pray for miraculous healing! Let us press together and let God be glorified.

Author Contact Page

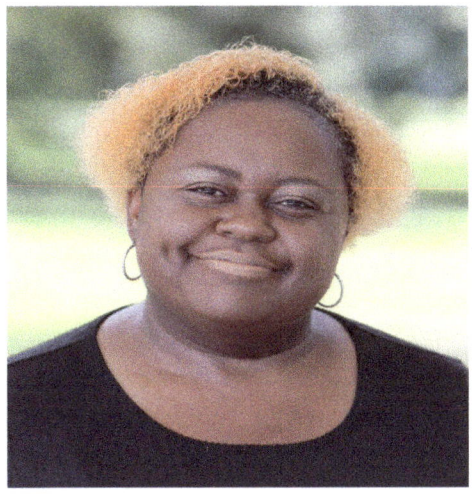

For more information address:
Yolawilliams40@gmail.com

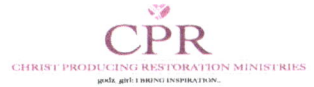

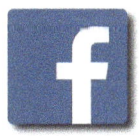 Christ Producing Restoration

 yagirl_yo_godzgirl

Milton Keynes UK
Ingram Content Group UK Ltd.
UKHW020339181123
432768UK00010B/264